The Gluten Free Solution - Learn How to Live a Gluten Free Life

Volume 1

Copyright information

Alon, Doron M.

The Gluten Free Solution - Learn How to Live a Gluten Free Life

—1st ed

ISBN: 978-0692594049

Printed in the United States of America

Cover image : #69831809 © adrenalinapura

Book Cover Design: Created by Doron M. Alon

doron@numinositypress.com

DEDICATION:
DEDICATED TO YOU

Disclaimer

By law, I need to add this statement. This book is for educational purposes only and does not claim to prevent or cure any disease. The advice in this book should not be construed as medical advice. Please seek advice from a professional if you have any health related issues.

By purchasing this book, you understand that results are not guaranteed. In light of this, you understand that in the unlikely event that this book does not work or causes harm in any area of your life, you agree that you do not hold Doron M. Alon, Numinosity Press Inc, its employees or affiliates liable for any damages you may experience or incur.

The Text is copyrighted 2015 by Numinosity Press Incorporated.

Introduction

Welcome to the first edition of The Gluten Free Series. A New Series dedicated to those who simply want to live a gluten free life without all the fuss and complication.

The interest in Gluten Free living has taken off in recent years due to the increasing number of people who have been diagnosed to have some form of gluten sensitivity. Although a gluten free lifestyle was made popular by the existence of an autoimmune condition called Celiac Disease, many have taken up the gluten free life style to improve their health in general.

In this volume of The Gluten Free Series, we will discuss what gluten is, the various conditions gluten causes for people who are sensitive to it, as well as common misconceptions about a gluten sensitivity and the gluten free lifestyle. We will also discuss ways to make transitioning to a gluten free life style easy. Like any radical change, it has to be done in a way that can be sustainable. For some, they have no choice, they must be gluten free while for others, it will be more for lifestyle change. This book will help both sides of the gluten spectrum.

Chapter 1: What is Gluten?

As I mentioned in the introduction, Gluten and its health implications has become the subject of intense focus over the last few years. Despite this, not many people know what Gluten is exactly. In this chapter, we will discuss what this maligned protein is and its natural characteristics.

The word gluten gives away much of what it is. In Latin, Gluten means glue. It is a protein ,not a carbohydrate like so many people think. Gluten is found in most grains but not all. Gluten is found in Rye, Barley and wheat, as well as other similar grains. If you have ever made bread or other recipes that require the making of dough, you have probably witnessed Gluten firsthand. Gluten gives that elastic feel to dough. It not only helps dough rise but it also gives breads and crusts that chewy consistency. It can't be denied, a chewy pizza crust is quite amazing and its all thanks to gluten.

Gluten is not only found in breads, but it is often found in a wide range of products such as Cosmetics, medications, skin products and other beauty products just to name a few. It is also in many packaged foods. It is all pervasive. We will discuss what to avoid on a gluten free lifestyle in a future chapter.

Gluten itself is not made of one single component, but rather it is a combination of Gliadin and a Glutenin, both proteins found in wheat and other cereal grains. These proteins form gluten proper. They are set together with the starchy parts and the endosperm of grain; or the inner part of a grain seed. Although Grains are considered carbohydrates, the gluten contain in the grain is a protein. 80% of the protein content of a wheat grain is gluten.

Gluten is often used as a protein alterative for people who are vegetarian and or vegan. Wheat gluten for example is used as a "faux meat". The most popular of these protein alternatives is a called Seitan. Seitan is quite an amazing product, it is by far the best faux meat on the market. Its versatility is quite amazing. Unfortunately, it is the worst thing you can have if you are trying to lead a gluten free lifestyle.

On the outset, it looks like a relatively benign protein, it almost sounds healthy. But for many people, it causes sustained discomfort and often debilitating health related issues. In the following chapters, I will briefly discuss Celiac disease and Gluten Sensitivity in general; they are not necessarily synonymous.

Chapter 2: Gluten Sensitivity

As I just mentioned, gluten sensitivity and celiac disease are not necessarily the same condition. Yes, Celiac disease is a condition brought on by gluten, it is much more severe than generalized gluten sensitivity. In this chapter we will discuss Gluten Sensitivity.

Although Celiac represents the face of gluten sensitivity, there are other conditions that are also tied to gluten sensitivity. These are often called Non-Celiac Gluten Sensitivity or NCGS for short.

Unfortunately, it is not particular easy to diagnose Non-Celiac gluten sensitivity with a test since there is no specific biomarker that can be used to diagnose it.   The best way to discern if you are gluten sensitive is to abstain from gluten for a period of time and see how you do.

Like Celiac and grain allergies in general, the common symptoms of gluten sensitivity are wide ranging. From gastrointestinal disturbances such as abdominal pain, constipation and on the flipside diarrhea as well as generalized bloating. Often over the counter medications are not very helpful for alleviating these symptoms. They might take the edge off, but nothing other than complete gluten abstinence can relieve these symptoms. Gluten sensitivity can also cause a wide range of generalized symptoms which include depression, numbness in the arms and legs, achy joints and muscles , anemia and what is called " foggy brain."

No one group of people is more susceptible to Non-Celiac Gluten Sensitivity than others. It seems to occur over a wide spectrum of individuals regardless of their medical histories. Although hints can be gleaned from personal history of food allergies and other tests to measure allergic reactions. Although these tests can be useful, it is still common practice to rule out celiac disease and wheat allergies by abstaining from gluten for a period of time. For people with Non-Celiac Gluten Sensitivity, abstinence will often resolve the issues within a few days to a few weeks.

For Scientific studies on Non-Celiac Gluten Sensitivity; please look at the following:

Mansueto, Pasquale; Seidita, Aurelio; D'Alcamo, Alberto; Carroccio, Antonio (2014). "Non-Celiac Gluten Sensitivity: Literature Review". *Journal of the American College of Nutrition* (Review) **33** (1): 39–54. doi:10.1080/07315724.2014.869996. ISSN 0731-5724. PMID 24533607.

Volta, Umberto; Caio, Giacomo; Tovoli, Francesco; De Giorgio, Roberto (2013). "Non-celiac gluten sensitivity: an emerging syndrome with many unsettled issues". *Italian Journal of Medicine* **8** (4): 225. doi:10.4081/itjm.2013.461. ISSN 1877-9352.

In the next chapter, we will discuss Celiac Disease.

Chapter 3: Celiac Disease

Unlike general gluten sensitivity, Celiac disease is a much more serious condition. About 1 in 133 people have this condition and it is often hereditary. Celiac disease, far beyond a gluten sensitivity, is an autoimmune disease in which the body is triggered by gluten and targets it as a toxic chemical. This process initiates a cascading and dysfunctional immune response that attacks the intestine, more specifically, the small intestine. In the small intestine, there are small fingerlike protrusions called Villi that help absorb nutrients. When a person has celiac disease, the immune system, triggered by gluten will attack the Villi. When this happens ,the body will slowly become deprived of vital nutrients for proper day-to-day functioning.

As I stated earlier, it seems to attack all population groups. It also appears that it can happen at any age. No one particular age category is predisposed to Celiac disease. It's an equal opportunity condition.

Short term Symptoms of Celiac Disease:

In the short term, the symptoms may seem rather broad and similar to plain gluten sensitivity such as: Bloating, diarrhea, fluctuations in weight, either gaining or losing, generalized weakness and fatigue , abdominal discomfort and in some cases it causes treatment-resistant depression also known as treatment-refractory depression.

Long term Symptoms of Celiac Disease:

In the long term, the symptoms can be far more acute. If left untreated it can predispose a person to other autoimmune diseases that can be fatal. Some of these include Diabetes, MS (Multiple Sclerosis) , Bone disorders such as osteoporosis, migraines, intestinal malignancies and epilepsy. Other symptoms can include miscarriages, infertility, itchy skin and rash and anemia amongst other things.

Celiac disease can also be A-symptomatic, which seems counterintuitive, but some people have been known to have Celiac disease and not have symptoms. Please note, the above symptoms are just a few. For the sake of brevity , I am just representing the most common ones. To see a more comprehensive list, please go to http://www.celiac.org (I am not associated with celiac.org or its affiliates) and find out more about the various symptoms.

Celiac Disease diagnosis:

Unlike general non-celiac gluten sensitivity, there are tests for Celiac disease. The most common test is called " tTG-IgA", if it comes back positive, then a biopsy of the lower intestine would be warranted to make the diagnosis definitive. The biopsy would show if the Villi are damaged or not. It is important to get tested WHEN you are going through symptoms so the test can pick up the antibodies. If you or a loved one thinks you might have Celiac Disease, please consult a physician and discuss your concerns with them. You may get a referral to a Gastroenterologist for further testing. if you do not have a primary care physician please to go http://www.celiac.org and they can provide a service that will help you find a physician specialist. (I am not associated with celiac.org or its affiliates)

If you are positive for Celiac disease, do not despair, there is an effective treatment that does not involve taking medication. The treatment is a Gluten Free Lifestyle. We will discuss what this entails in a future chapter. But before I get into that, I want to cover wheat allergy and how it differs from gluten sensitivity and celiac disease. They are often confused.

Chapter 4: Wheat Allergy

One of the most common misconceptions is that a wheat allergy is synonymous with Celiac disease and Gluten sensitivity. One thing they do have in common is that they activate the immune system. They do this in different ways and that is what makes them so different.

As I stated in the previous chapter, Celiac disease is when the immune system malfunctions because it treats gluten as a poison. When it does this, it causes the immune system to attack the lower intestine. With a wheat allergy, something all together happens.

Whereas Celiac is a malfunction of the immune system, a wheat allergy is an OVERREACTION of the immune system. Unlike Celiac disease that can progress overtime before it becomes symptomatic; an Allergic response is almost immediate or within a few short hours. When proteins, starches or other components in wheat are introduced into the system, an allergic reaction such as swelling, rashes, hives and itching can occur. If the Allergy is more acute, it can affect breathing and cause fainting. If it is very bad, an allergy can be fatal. These symptoms are sudden onset and are often treated with anti-histamines.

Another difference is that a person with a wheat allergy may not necessarily have allergies to other grains; approximately 20% of people who do have wheat allergies can be allergic to other grains as well. With Celiac disease and gluten sensitivity, almost all other grains will also be a problem. That is because A Wheat Allergy can be an allergy to other proteins or starches in the wheat itself ; whereas Celiac is specific to the Gluten Protein found in wheat and other grains. We will discuss grains that do not have gluten in a future chapter.

Another stark difference is that some people who are allergic to Wheat can get triggered by exercising a few hours after eating it. This might sound rather odd, but Some people do get what is called Wheat dependent , exercise induced anaphylaxis. The exercise hastens or worsens the immune response to the Wheat allergen, often this triggering is fatal. This is not found amongst gluten sensitive conditions.

As a side note: Generally speaking, Wheat allergies are mostly found in children and are outgrown by the age of 3 or 4. **HOWEVER, adults can be allergic as well.** Celiac and Gluten sensitivity can occur at any time and aren't **generally** the types of conditions that are outgrown overtime. If anything, if left untreated will worsen . In saying that, I would like to mention that although It is exceedingly rare that someone would outgrow Celiac or Gluten Sensitivity, it has happened. A study in the Journal "Gut" was published in October of 2007 and reported children outgrowing it as they grew into adulthood. But again, that is exceedingly rare.

In the next chapter, I will discuss which grains should be avoided if you want to live a gluten free lifestyle.

Chapter 5: Foods To Avoid If You Want To Get Rid Of Gluten

We live in a gluten-filled world, there is no doubt about that. Admittedly, there are quite a few things you will need to look out for, but in this day and age, living a gluten free life is easier than ever.   In this chapter, we will discuss what YOU CANNOT have if you have Gluten sensitivity or Celiac disease.

Here is a basic list of foods you **can't** eat. This is just a starter list, I am sure you there are a few more foods, but for now, this should be enough to get you started on your path to a Gluten Free lifestyle.

The number one culprit is wheat. The thing is wheat has various derivative products that also contain gluten.

Grains to avoid:

Wheat (Even if a label says wheat free, it does not mean it is gluten free, please check the labels carefully)

Einkorn Wheat

Durum

Kamut also known as Khorasan wheat

Emmer

Graham

Semolina

Farro

Spelt

Farina

Triticale

Rye

Barley

Brewer's Yeast

Malt: Malt can come in various forms such as . Malt Vinegar, Malted Barley Flour, Malt flavorings, Malted Milk also known as Malted Milkshakes, Malt Syrup, Malt extract.

Wheat Starch: In some instances gluten has been removed from the starch, but you must check the label to make sure.

Here is a partial list of popular foods that contain gluten .

Breads of various kinds such as Donuts, Croissants, Bagels, various flatbreads, rolls, potato bread , cornbread

Cracks of various kinds.

Cookies

Brownies

breadcrumbs and croutons

Cakes and pie crusts

Cereals . Generally speaking most cereals on the market contain gluten . Some will state definitively that they are gluten free and some will not. The ones that do not need to be check closely. You may still be able to eat them, but be on the lookout for favoring agents such as Malt. Although they may contain gluten free grains, they may still have gluten from flavoring agents.

Flour Tortillas (Corn Tortillas are safe)

Pastas and noodles: of various kinds including Gnocchi, Raviolis, Manicotti, Couscous , dumplings. There are, of course several other kinds of pasta. In the noodle category we have Soba, chow mien, lo mien, ramen, udon and egg noodles. If the noodles are made of rice than they are gluten free.

Typical Breakfast foods that contain gluten are : Biscuits, Pancakes, Crepes, Waffles and French toast.

Sauces ,Soups and Salad dressings: This category is by the far the trickiest of them all. Moist sauce, soups and dressings are made with thinking agents that more often than not contain gluten . Please read the labels before buying these items. **Soy Sauce is a hidden source of Gluten, but must be verified before purchasing. Some do not contain gluten.**

Poultry that is self basting.

Meats that are pre-seasoned: Can often contain hidden sources of gluten. Label should be checked.

Sports bars, energy bars , granola bars and candy bars: Always check the labels on these, often they are packed with gluten containing agents.

Fried foods: These are tricky too. Often the batter is made of a wheat product such as flour.

Potato chips : Often then are seasoned with Gluten containing agents. Please check labels. There are a few gluten free varieties that are excellent.

Deli and processed meats: Often they are processed with a flavoring agent that contains gluten. Make sure to read the label carefully. Although its a meat, the processing might taint it with gluten.

Meat substitutes or " Faux meat" : The most obvious one is Seitan which is straight wheat gluten. Imitation seafood, imitation bacon , vegi burgers and the like MUST be examined carefully. Often these will contain wheat derived protein. This category really requires your full attention before you buy them.

Alcoholic Drinks:_ Non-distilled drinks such as Malt drinks, lagers, Beer and ales do contain gluten and should be avoided.

Supplements (vitamins, minerals, protein shakes, herbals): Not all vitamins and supplements are gluten free. You must check those labels very closely.

Medications: Not all medications are gluten free. you must check those labels very closely. Often they contain filler, inactive ingredients and coatings that may contain gluten. Ask your pharmacist for help with all your OTC and prescription medications.

Makeup, lip balms and the like: Often they are made of gluten containing products and are at risk of being accidently ingested.

This, of course, is not an exhausted list but one to get you started. I know it seems like a lot, but there are many alternatives which we will get into in future chapters. But before we finish this chapter I would like to point out a possible area of concern... Mostly, cross contamination. You might buy and eat gluten free products but it doesn't mean it can't be cross contaminated with gluten containing agents. We will go over briefly a few places to look out for that may contain cross-contaminating potential.

Toaster ovens: Often toaster ovens are the number one place that a cross contamination can occur since it is used to toast gluten containing products. Make sure they are well cleaned. If you can, get one for yourself if you live with others who do not have gluten issues.

Fryers: Deep fryers may contain gluten since most batters are made of flour and this contain gluten.

Containers that may have been shared with gluten containing food.

Flour Sifting and handling instruments

Condiment jars and containers: If someone drips bread into them or a crump gets into them, the condiment may be contaminated with a gluten containing agent.

Pizza Parlors that have a gluten free variety: Although a pizza place may serve gluten free pizza, they may also serve regular pizza and this causes a serious contamination risk. Best to look for places that are gluten free.

I will get into some strategies you can use to reduce contamination in your home in an upcoming chapter.

I know that it seems that you are very limited as to what you can have if you are gluten sensitivity or have celiac disease, but it isn't as bad as it seems. There are plenty alternatives. Yes, you are limited to some degree, but as you will see in the following chapters, you have more than enough variety to make a gluten free lifestyle a viable choice for you.

Chapter 6: Foods You Can Have

The number 1 food group that people with Celiac and Gluten Sensitivities miss the most are, well, grains. After all, grains are in all of our favorite foods such Pizza, bread, pasta , cake, you name it. All the comfort foods. All is not lost though. Nowadays there are plenty of brands out there that make great gluten free alternatives. I will list the brands in a separate chapter . In this chapter I will focus specifically on foods you can eat. And YES, YOU CAN HAVE PIZZA, BREAD, PASTA AND CAKE. You will just need to use gluten free grains. We will get into those in this chapter.

Basically, you can eat anything that doesn't contain gluten , which is quite a lot actually.

Here is a basic list of foods you can eat. This is just a starter list, I am sure you there are many more foods, but for now, this should be enough to get you started on your path to a Gluten Free lifestyle.

The safest foods:

Dairy: Milk, Margarine, Cream, Butter and cheese

All meats and poultry

All fruits and Vegetables , including dried (Please Keep in mind that Barley Grass and Wheat Grass are gluten free, however, their respective seeds contain gluten so please proceed with caution, not all establishments handle these properly and the risk of gluten contamination is possible)

All fish and Seafood

Legumes , beans and nuts are also gluten free

Eggs

Sugar

Honey and Molasses

** The only time you should be careful with fruit and nuts is if they are processed ,canned or dried. Sometimes the processing may contain elements that contain gluten. So the labels should be read closely.

Now to the good part.

Gluten Free Grains , flours and starchy foods:

Nut flours (Perfect for making gluten free breads and other "bready foods" and crusts)

Rice

Oats (Please be mindful since most oats are processed with the same equipment as wheat and other gluten containing grains, please be sure the packaging specifically states gluten free)

Cassava also known as Arrowroot, Manioc, Tapioca

Yucca

Corn (And Yes even Corn Tortillas when not exposed to flour)

Chia seeds

Soy beans

Flax

Potato

Teff (Although this does contain a kind of gluten, the gluten in Teff does not have the Gliadin, thus making it safe for a gluten free lifestyle)

Amaranth

Sorghum

buckwheat aka KASHA

Quinoa

Millet

To be on the safe side and to exercise maximum caution, please read the labels to make sure these products are truly gluten free. Sometimes the processing and the harvesting of these grains could expose them to gluten containing grains. Remember, just because a product is wheat free does not mean it is gluten free. Check the labels well.

Alcoholic Drinks: In general, hard distilled drinks such as liquor, vodka and hard ciders are gluten free because the distillation process removes the gluten.

Non-alcoholic drinks: Most sports drinks, REAL FRUIT juices and sodas are gluten free.

Supplements (vitamins, minerals, protein shakes, herbals): As stated in the previous chapter, not all vitamins and supplements are gluten free. you must check those labels very closely.

Medications: As stated in the previous chapter, not all medications are gluten free. You must check those labels very closely. Often they contain filler, inactive ingredients and coatings that may contain gluten. Ask your pharmacist for help with all your OTC and prescription medications.

If you don't have the time to prepare any of the ingredients above, like I mentioned, there are TONS of gluten free substitutes. If you have a Trader Joes around you, they have a gluten free foods to die for. There are also several gluten free breads as well. Living Gluten Free can be done. I'll get into various brands in a future chapter. I will also give you a few recipes to get you started using the ingredients above. You'll see that it can be pretty easy to start and maintain a gluten free lifestyle.

Chapter 7: How To Avoid Cross-Contamination At Home

You may live with others who do not have celiac disease and so you will need to make some changes so you don't contaminate your gluten free food with their gluten containing foods.

Here are a few tips:

When you are shopping make sure to purchase gluten free products a that are not sharing the same bins or shelves that contain gluten containing food.

As I stated In a previous chapter, having your own toaster oven would be most ideal.

When dealing with condiments, When possible, buy 2 of each item so that you can be safe that your item has not been contaminated. For example, if you like peanut butter or other condiments; Have your own jar so as to minimize the risk that someone might have put a bread containing knife or spoon in your jar or container. Label your jar as gluten free or put your name on it.

When using gluten free flour, place it in a contain and cover it and place it in another cabinet so it won't get contaminated by other , gluten containing flours.

Clean your counter tops and cutting boards very often to minimize contaminating with gluten containing agents.

When using spices, get the pure blends and not the blended one that can contain gluten contamination. Check the label closely.

When storing your gluten free foods, place them on top of the gluten containing ones if you don't have extra storage space. This will minimize any thing falling out of the gluten containing foods and contaminating yours.

Labeling your food and cleaning your shared kitchen space is vital for your gluten free life style to work. By following some of the tips above, you can lower your risk of gluten contamination.

Chapter 8: Eating Out Gluten Free

Eating out while being gluten free can pose some challenges. Not all restaurants have gluten free options. BUT that doesn't mean you can't enjoy eating out. It just takes a bit more leg work.

Here are a few tips on how to make it work for you:

If you know which restaurant you are going to check their website or give them a call. They may have a gluten free menu or at least a few gluten free options available. Nowadays, quite a few places exist that offer gluten free options.

Once you identify these options ask them how these are prepared. Is there a risk of cross contamination?

Try to avoid pizza parlors and bakeries that bake gluten containing breads, there is a high risk of contamination. There are, however, gluten free bakeries popping up. I'd do a search and see if any have opened. I know, in my neighborhood a gluten free bakery popped up and it is always packed.

Before ordering do let them know of your gluten sensitivity

The best thing you can do is always use your best judgment. If you feel a place might not be suitable, you should skip it. Your best bet is to search for places near you. I am sure you will find an establishment. They are popping up quite frequently. IF there aren't any, you'll need to order dishes that you know are gluten free by default. In the next chapter will discuss common myths and misconceptions about gluten free. After that we will discuss brands and recipes.

Chapter 9: Common Myths About A Gluten Free Lifestyle

Like many subjects there will always be notions and ideas that are downright false. This is no different for nutrition, especially as it pertains to gluten free living. In this chapter, we will debunk some of these myths once and for all. These myths seem to persist despite evidence to the contrary. I am hoping you will get some clarity after you read this chapter.

Myth 1: Gluten free is low carb. One of the most persistent myths about gluten free food is that it is low carb. It's not low carb at all. I think the confusion arises because gluten is found in grain. And grain is a carbohydrate. Gluten is simply a protein within grain and itself is not a carbohydrate. As you saw in previous chapters , much of the gluten free foods are , in fact, carbohydrates.

Myth 2: All wheat products are forbidden for you. This is not true even if it seems counterintuitive since Gluten is derived from Wheat. However, if the gluten is removed from the grain it will make that grain safe. Gluten can be removed from wheat and other grains thus making it safe for consumption. For example, wheat based glucose syrup can be safe if the gluten is removed in the processing.

Myth 3: Vinegar is packed with gluten. Vinegar is generally gluten free since the production of vinegar involves a distillation process that removes the gluten from the product. Even if the vinegar is made out of wheat. **<u>But be careful, look for distilled vinegar NOT Fermented .</u>**

Myth 4: Most if not all prescriptions contain gluten containing binding agents and fillers. There is no doubt that many do. But generally speaking this is not true. Many are gluten free. If you are concerned, please speak to your pharmacist. If they can't help you or if you want further confirmation you can look up some popular drugs for gluten at www.glutenfreedrugs.com.

Myth 5: Gluten Free Food is always healthier. I know it is counterintuitive of me to state this but gluten free food is not necessarily healthier for a person who doesn't have gluten issues.

Myth 6: Being Gluten Free is almost always good for digestive health. This is true pretty much for those with gluten sensitivity. Otherwise it has not been proven to cause much disturbance for people who do not have gluten issues.

Myth 7: Gluten free food is bland. Like any food, it's all in the preparation. I have had outstanding gluten free dishes and breads. As I stated earlier, trader Joes has gluten free food that is excellent.

Myth 8: Gluten containing grains are GMO (Genetically modified) . Truth is, the gluten content of any given grain is mutually exclusive from how it is grown. Both Gluten containing and gluten free products can both be GMO. The only way to know is to look at the labels. Some products will tell you if they are truly GMO or GMO free. When in doubt, a health food grocery store would be the best place to go to find GMO free products.

Myth 9: I have no symptoms thus I don't have Celiac Disease. If you have been diagnosed with celiac but seem to have few no or no symptoms doesn't mean you have been cured of Celiac disease. Symptoms can come later. This is not like an allergy that symptoms pop up right away.

Myth 10: Wheat-fed animals meant for human consumption contain gluten. Absolutely not, there is no way for gluten to hide in the muscle tissue. Meat is gluten free whether the animal eats grass or wheat.

Myth 11: All my symptoms are because of Gluten Sensitivity or Celiac disease. Last time we all checked, we are still human and susceptible to the same illness whether gluten sensitive or not :)

These are just a few myths, there are several more. In the next chapter I will give alist of a few brands that are either completely gluten free or make gluten free foods. You will see that this list is quite extensive.

Chapter 10: Gluten Free Brands

In this chapter I will list quite a few brands that make gluten free foods. Some carry gluten free exclusively and some simply have gluten free options. I will separate them by category for ease reference.

Baby Food Brands:

Baby Mum-Mum

Beech-Nut

Happy Baby

Little Duck Organics

Plum Organics

Meat And Poultry:

Aidells

Applegate

Bar S

Bell and Evans

Carl Buddig & Company

Coleman Natural

Dietz & Watson

Golden Platter All Natural

Fra Mani

Habbersett Scrapple

Hans All Natural

Harvestland Brand

Ian's

Perdue

Rocky Mountain Organic Meats

Sabrett

Smithfield

Thumanns

Tyson Foods

Bagels, Baked goods, Breads:

Aleia's Gluten Free Foods

Allie's GF Goodies

Bites of Bliss

Bonnievilles

Canyon Bakehouse

Chocorice

Cookies...for me?

Crave Right

Deanna's Gluten Free Bakery

Doodles Cookies

Dr. Lucy's

EatPastry

El's Gluten Free Cookies

Ener-G Foods

Enjoy Life Foods-Cookies

Flax4Life

Glenny's

Gluten Free Houston

Glutino

Go Big Oat!

HomeFree

Ian's

Jensen's Bread and Bakeries

Joans GF Great Bakes

Joey's Home Bakery

Kinnikinnick Foods

Licious Organics

Liz Lovely

Maple Grove Farms

Mariposa Artisan-Crafted Gluten Free - Oakland

Marlas Sweet Treats

MI-DEL Cookies

Mina's Purely Divine

Molly B's Gluten-Free Kitchen

Montana Monster Munchies

Moon Rabbit foods

Nu-World Foods

O'Doughs

PatsyPie

Penn Street Bakery

Pillsbury

R.W. Bakers

Rudi's Gluten Free Bakery

Savory Foods

Schar USA

Sweet Megan Baking Company

The Bites Company

Udi's Gluten Free Foods

Whole Foods Market

Wholly Wholesome

Wholly Wholesome - Pizza Dough

Cereals:

Barbara's Cereal

Bob's Red Mill

Chex

Cream of Rice

Earth's Supergrains

Enjoy Life Foods-Breakfast Cereal

Freedom Foods

Glutenfreeda Foods

Jessica's Natural Foods

Orgran

Shiloh Farms

Gluten Free Flours

Bay State Milling

Bloomfield Farms

Bob's Red Mill

GF Jules

GloryBee Foods

Hodgson Mill

LifeField

Meister's Gluten Free Mixtures

Mr. Ritts

Nu Life Market

Nu-World Foods

Prairie Star

Salad Dressing and Sauces

5th Sun Specialties

Annies Naturals

Ass Kickin Sauces

Bone Suckin' Sauce

Bove's Pasta Sauces

Frank's Redhot

Gone Native

Green Mountain Gringo

Heinz Classico Red

Kikkoman Sales USA, Inc.

Maple Grove Farms

Maxwells Kitchen

Mrs. Lauralicious

Nacheez

Organic Nectars

Pace Sauce

Riega Cheese Sauce Mixes

San-J International

Simply Boulder

Sophia's Gourmet Foods

Stubb's Legendary Kitchen

Tabasco

Three Acre Kitchen

Wing-Time Buffalo Wing Sauce

Gluten Free Alcoholic Beverages:

Angry Orchard

Chopin Vodkas

Daura

Devotion Vodka

Disaronno

Dogfish Head Tweason' Ale

Hiram Walker

Krome Vodka

Lakefront Brewery - New Grist

Lyle Style

Omission Beer

Redbridge Beer

Gluten Free Juices

ALO Drink

Buddy Fruit

Caribbean Passion

Fox Barrel Cider

Hawaiian Punch

Jamba Juice

Langers Juices

Minute Maid

Mott's

Newman's Own

Old Orchard Juices

Organic Avenue

Sobe Beverages

Tropicana

V8

Welch's

Gluten Free Milk and Milk Substitutions

8th Continent Soy Milk

Almond Fresh

Augason Farms

Lactaid

Living Harvest -Tempt Hempmilk

Meyenberg Goat Milk

NadaMoo!

Vitasoy Lite Plus

Gluten Free Ice Teas

Bigelow Tea

High Country Kombucha

Snapple

Sobe Beverages

Gluten Free Hot Chocolate

Burnham & Mills

Gluten Free Energy Drinks

Columbia Gorge Organic

Gatorade

Golazo

GT's Kombucha

Perfect Fit by Tone It Up

Red Bull

Gluten Free Soft Drinks

7up

Canada Dry

Coca Cola

Dr. Pepper

Mountain Dew

Orange Crush

Pepsi Cola

RC Cola

Reeds Sodas

Schweppes

Zevia Soda

Chocolates and Sweets

Alter Eco

Angell Organic Candy Bars

Betty Lou's

Cadbury

Candy Tree

ChocAlive

Coco Polo/YC Chocolatier

Dove Chocolate

Enjoy Life Foods-Chocolate Bars

Froose

KatySweet Confectioners

Miles of Chocolate

Organic Nectars

Righteously Raw Bars

Spangler Candy

Sweet Pete's

Cosmetics

Afterglow Cosmetics

Ahava

Andrea Rose Personal Basics

Arbonne International

Bare Minerals Foundation

Bronze Buffer

Derma E

Devita

Dr. Hauschka

Ecco Bella

Gabriel Cosmetics

Gluten Freed Skin Care

Juice Beauty - The Organic Solution

Kiss My Face

Larenim Mineral

Logona Natural Body Care

Mineral Fusion

NARS Cosmetics

PRIIA Cosmetics

Pur Skn

Red Apple Lipstick

Sappho Cosmetics

Sibu Beauty

Synergy Hair

Ulta Beauty

Vapour Organic Beauty

Pasta

Ancient Harvest

Annie Chun's

Explore Asian

Gia Russa

Hodgson Mill

Leo's Gluten Free

Namaste Foods

Orgran

Road's End Organics

Ronzoni Gluten Free

Schar USA

Taste Up Foods

Pizza

7 Sisters Gluten-Free

Better 4U Foods

Bloomfield Farms

Dad's Gluten-Free Pizza Crust

Gillian's foods

Kinnikinnick Foods

Pizza Fusion

Schar USA

Still Riding Pizza

Trader Joes

Wholly Wholesome - Pizza Dough

Z Pizza

Soups

Dr. McDougall's Right Foods

Gluten Free Cafe

Health Valley

Pacific Farms

Pacific Natural Foods

Progresso

San-J International

Swanson

The Organic Gourmet

Wolfgang Puck

Gluten Free Rice and Grains

Alter Eco

Better Bean

Konriko

Lotus Foods

Nu Life Market

As you can see, there are dozens upon dozens of companies that create gluten free foods. If you have gluten sensitivity or Celiac diseases you will find the above brands will cover most , if not all of your needs quite well. In the next chapter I will supply you with a few recipes you can try that are gluten free....Enjoy.

Chapter 11: Gluten Recipes

In this chapter I will provide you with 5 super easy gluten free recipes that you will love. Please stay tuned for Volume 3 and 4 of this series. In those volumes I will supply you many more recipes. Hope you enjoy these.

Bread Recipe:

Gluten Free Focaccia Bread: I personally love Focaccia bread and this recipe is as close to the gluten variety as you can get without the gluten. Enjoy.

Ingredients

3 cups of Bobs Red Mill Gluten Free all purpose Flour

1.5 teaspoons Xanthan Gum

1 teaspoon kosher salt

2 tablespoons of sugar

2 packets of yeast

2 cups warm water,

2 teaspoons olive oil

Olive Oil

Fresh rosemary (optional, but if you want the authtic feel you should use it)

Sea salt

Instructions

Preheat Your oven to 400° Fahrenheit.

Rub or spray the olive oil in a cake pan.

Mix the dry ingredients using the regular beater.

Add the warm water and olive oil and make sure they are mixed well. Scrape bottom and sides of bowl, beaters. Dough should be a little soft and slightly tacky.

Prepare the warm water in a bowl. Place dough in the pan and wet your hand in the water bowl, make sure it is not dripping wet so shake off the excess as best you can. Spread the dough out to the sides of the pan. You may wet your hands again so the dough doesn't stick.

Cover the dough and let it rise in a warm place for 30-40 minutes.

Sprinkle olive oil or spray olive oil over the top of the bread. Make sure not to put too much, just lightly. You dont want the bread to get too oily.

Add the rosemary and sea salt or whatever topping you like

Bake breads for 20-30 minutes. Generally, when golden brownish areas appear over its surface that means it's about done.

Remove from pan and let the bread cool down a bit.

Cut with a serrated knife the way that you like it.

There you have it, Gluten Free **Focaccia Bread.**

Pizza Recipe:

THE SAUCE

28-ounce can whole peeled tomatoes, MAKE SURE TO DRAIN THEM

1 tablespoon virgin olive oil

1 garlic clove, minced well.

1 teaspoon dried oregano

3/4 teaspoon salt

1/4 teaspoon pepper optional (I am not a pepper person myself)

THE CHEESE

8 ounces shredded mozzarella cheese

THE CRUST

16 ounces America's Bobs Red Mill Gluten Free all purpose Flour

1/2 cup plus 1 tablespoon almond flour

2 1/2 teaspoons baking powder

1.5 teaspoons salt

1 teaspoon yeast

2 1/2 cups warm water (100 degrees Fahrenheit)

1/4 cup vegetable oil

Olive oil spray

Instructions for the Sauce:

Place all the ingredients in a food processer and make sure to process until smooth.

Instructions for the Crust:

Mix all the dry ingredients well, preferably with a stand mixer.

Slowly add the water and oil until it is well incorporated with the dry ingredients.

Pick up the mixing pace until the dough is sticky , something resembling a very thick batter. In a stand mixer it should be about 5-7 minutes.

Remove the dough and cover with plastic wrap until the dough puffs up. It won't rise per -se but should puff up and become bubbly. Let it stand for 1.5 hours.

Line 2 baking sheets, make sure they have rimms. Line them with parchment paper and spray on the oil liberally. Now spread the dough. Spray the top of the dough with oil as well.

Press out the dough as thick as you like but make sure the edges are thicker by about 1/4 - 1/2 inches. You can make it as thick as you like.

Place the 2 lined baking sheets in the oven at 350 degrees. Bake the dough until it is just about turning brown, this should take about 40-45 minutes. You don't want to cook the dough through just yet.

Once browned, remove the dough trays and let it cool down a bit, preferably about an hour.

Now you are ready to add topping and bake your pizza.

Set the baking stone in the oven and bring the oven to 500 degrees.

Transfer one of the pizza crusts to a pizza peel and ladle out some sauce. As much as you want but I'd suggest 1/2 cup so it doesn't get soggy. Spread the sauce evenly leaving a little bit of room at the crust edge.

Sprinkle the mozzarella sauce on the pizza.

Place Pizza on the stone and bake for 12 minute or so until the cheese bubbles and the crust turns golden brown.

Let cool and serve :)

Banana Pancakes:

Ingredients:
1 ripe banana. Not too ripe, just partially
1 large egg
Butter

Cinnamon
Honey (Optional for topping)
Nuts (Optional for topping if you like)

Instructions:

Place the Banana in a bowl and Mash the Banana with a fork until there are no clumps.

Then add the egg and beat it into the banana mash.

Put the butter in the skillet (as much butter as you like)

Turn your stove on to medium high. make sure the butter is completely covering the surface of the skillet.

Pour the batter into pan. This should make about 3 pancakes.

Sprinkle some cinnamon on the pancakes, let them brown and then flip them over. Cook then until they are golden and make sure centers are cooked.

Serve on a plate and add your toppings :)

Delicious right?

2 more recipes

http://recipes.glutenfreeresourcedirectory.com/uid/79af8ef6-85fd-45f3-ad56-f5d8be179da7/

Conclusion

Well, there you have it. As you can see, having Gluten issues is not the end of the world. Yes, you might need to deny yourself certain things but as you can see, there are many alternatives. We are lucky to live in a time where we can find so many alternatives to common food items. The best part in all this is that while you become mindful of foods that have gluten in them you also become mindful of food in general. Looking at labels create a habit and a mindset that can allow you to make better food choices in general, outside of just monitoring for gluten. Many people I know who are gluten sensitive or have celiac disease are now eating healthier in general despite the gluten issues. So no matter how you slice it, whether you are gluten sensitive or have celiac disease, this gives you an opportunity to really revamp the way that you eat. I see that as a huge plus.

Stay tuned for more books in this series. The following are forthcoming:

Book 2: Drop the Gluten, Drop The Weight.

Book 3: The Gluten Free Bread Making Cookbook: 20 Gluten Free Bread Recipes Your Whole Family Will Love.

Book 4: 20 Gluten Free Comfort food recipes

Go to www.glutenfreeseries.com to find out more.

About The Author

Doron Alon is a bestselling author of 50 books, in 6 different genres and is founder of Numinosity Press Inc.

Before he became an author and teacher, Doron majored in Business and Psychology, spending several years as an Entrepreneur, Wall Street Consultant and Healthcare Analyst. During that whole time, he pursued his intellectual and spiritual passions, leading him to the life that he leads today... One of teaching and service.

Now he writes on a wide variety of topics including History, Self-help, Self-Publishing, Spirituality and health related topics. Doron's background and 24 years of experience in meditation training, Meridian tapping (also known as E.F.T), Subliminal Messaging and other modalities has made him a much sought after expert in the self help and spirituality fields. He is also a up-and-coming expert in the self publishing field and health related topics. His conversational writing style and his ability to take complex topics and make them easily accessible has gained him popularity in the genres that he writes for. As he says " Translating esoteric topics and making them easy to understand" is his area of expertise.

Resources And References

Gluten Intolerance Group; www.gluten.net

Celiac Disease Foundation; www.celiac.org

Celiac Sprue Association-USA; www.csaceliacs.org

Canadian Celiac Association; www.celiac.ca

Gluten-Free Living; www.glutenfreeliving.com